FROM BACHELOR TO DAD

Navigating the Journey of First-Time Fatherhood

Robert D. Streeter

Table of contents

Preparing for Fatherhood

Pregnancy and Birth

Newborn Care

Sleep and Sleep Training

Feeding and Nutrition

Health and Safety

Developmental Milestones

Parenting Roles and Relationships

Financial Planning

Emotional Support

Father-Child Bonding

Discipline and Boundaries

Parenting Styles

Preparing for Future Stages

Self-Care

Community and Resources

Balancing Work and Parenting

Travelling with a Baby

Creating Memories

Conclusion

Preparing for Fatherhood

Becoming a first-time dad is a life-altering experience filled with excitement, anticipation, and, of course, a touch of anxiety. As you stand on the threshold of fatherhood, a whirlwind of emotions and questions may consume your thoughts. Rest assured, you are not alone in this journey. Countless men before you have embarked on this path, each with their unique stories, challenges, and joys. In this guide, we'll explore the incredible journey of becoming a first-time dad, from the initial moments of discovering the pregnancy to the profound responsibilities and joys that await.

Fatherhood is a profound and transformative journey that begins with the birth of a child. It is a role that has evolved significantly over the years, moving beyond traditional stereotypes to encompass a wide range of responsibilities and emotions.The essence of fatherhood, its evolving nature, and the importance of a father's presence in a child's life.

Historically, the role of a father was often limited to being the provider and protector of the family. However, societal norms and expectations have shifted, allowing fathers to embrace a more involved and nurturing role in their children's lives. This transformation has been driven by various factors, including changing gender roles, increased awareness of the benefits of involved fathering, and a greater emphasis on shared parenting responsibilities.

Today's fathers are no longer confined to the stereotype of distant and stoic figures. They actively engage in

caregiving, bonding, and emotional support for their children. Modern fathers change diapers, attend parent-teacher conferences, cook meals, and participate in bedtime routines. This active involvement not only strengthens the father-child relationship but also contributes significantly to a child's development.

One of the most critical aspects of fatherhood is the opportunity for fathers to build strong emotional bonds with their children. These bonds are nurtured through quality time spent together, such as playing games, sharing stories, and offering guidance. A father's presence and active participation provide children with a sense of security and support, which is essential for their emotional and social development.

Fathers also serve as essential role models for their children, teaching them values, ethics, and life skills. Children often look up to their fathers as examples of how to navigate the world. A responsible and loving father can instill confidence, resilience, and a sense of purpose in their offspring.

Pregnancy and Birth

The journey begins with the thrilling announcement of pregnancy and culminates in the awe-inspiring miracle of childbirth. As a first-time dad, here's what you can expect during this extraordinary adventure.

The journey of pregnancy starts with the joyous revelation that you and your partner are expecting. That positive pregnancy test brings forth a mix of emotions, from excitement to a touch of anxiety. You're now responsible for nurturing a new life, and the anticipation of meeting your child for the first time is overwhelming.

As the weeks progress, you'll witness incredible changes in your partner's body and emotions. Pregnancy is a time of growth, both for the baby and for your connection as a couple. You'll share in the milestones, from the first ultrasound image that reveals your baby's tiny heartbeat to feeling those initial flutters and kicks.

Your role as a first-time dad is crucial during pregnancy. Attend prenatal classes together, accompany your partner to doctor's appointments, and be her source of emotional support. Learn about the stages of pregnancy, and engage in open communication to better understand her needs and experiences.

In the months leading up to the birth, you'll likely find yourself engaged in a flurry of nesting activities. Assemble baby furniture, decorate the nursery, and pack the hospital bag. These preparations build excitement and ensure you're ready when the big day arrives.

Childbirth itself is a monumental moment. As a first-time dad, you'll be there to offer encouragement, hold her hand, and provide unwavering support. Witnessing the strength and determination of your partner during labour is a humbling experience. The sounds of labour pains, the rush to the hospital, and the anticipation in the delivery room are moments etched into your memory forever.

The most extraordinary part of this journey is the moment you meet your child for the first time. The overwhelming love and sense of responsibility that wash over you are indescribable. As you hold your newborn in your arms, you'll be filled with awe and gratitude.

Bringing your baby home marks the beginning of a new chapter as a family. As a first-time dad, you'll take on diaper duty, share midnight feedings, and become a master of soothing techniques. These shared experiences deepen your bond with your partner and strengthen your connection with your child.

Parenthood is a continual learning experience. You'll celebrate every milestone, from the first smile to the first steps. Through sleepless nights and moments of frustration, you'll discover an enduring wellspring of love and patience within yourself.

The journey of pregnancy and childbirth as a first-time dad is a profound and transformative experience. It's a journey filled with anticipation, support, and profound moments of wonder. Embrace each step, and cherish the bond you'll form with your partner and your child as you embark on this extraordinary adventure together.

Newborn Care

As you welcome your newborn into the world, one of the most important roles you'll take on is that of a caregiver. Newborn care can seem daunting at first, but with some guidance and preparation, you'll be well-equipped to ensure your baby's well-being and create lasting memories in these precious early weeks.

In the whirlwind of emotions that follow childbirth, the initial days with your newborn are a time of bonding and adjustment.Right after birth, spend quality time holding your baby skin-to-skin. This close contact promotes bonding, regulates the baby's temperature, and provides comfort.

Whether you choose to breastfeed or formula-feed, your baby's nourishment is a top priority. If your partner is breastfeeding, support her with patience and encouragement. If you're formula-feeding, follow the recommended guidelines for preparation and feeding.

Get ready for frequent diaper changes! Keep a stock of diapers, wipes, and a changing station ready. Remember to clean gently and apply diaper cream to prevent diaper rash.
As the days progress, you'll find yourself establishing routines for feeding and soothing your baby
Newborns often feed every 2-3 hours. Pay attention to your baby's cues for hunger and fullness. Burp your baby after each feeding to prevent gas discomfort.
Babies can get fussy for various reasons. Try swaddling, rocking, singing, or gentle shushing to comfort your little one. Sometimes, a pacifier can be soothing.

Encourage tummy time when your baby is awake and supervised. This helps develop neck and upper body strength.
Follow the recommended schedule of paediatrician visits and vaccinations. Keep

track of growth milestones and any concerns you may have.

Be cautious with bath time. Use lukewarm water and mild baby soap, and always support your baby's head and neck.Keep the umbilical cord stump clean and dry. It will naturally fall off within a few weeks.

Remember that bonding with your newborn is a two-way street. Spend quality time together, talking, singing, and making eye contact. Skin-to-skin cuddles are an excellent way to strengthen your connection.

Don't forget about self-care. Caring for a newborn can be exhausting, so ensure you get enough rest and seek help from family and friends when needed. Communicate openly with your partner about your feelings and share responsibilities.

Becoming a first-time dad is a remarkable journey filled with love and learning. Embrace the challenges and joys of newborn care, and cherish these precious moments as your baby grows. By providing love, care, and a safe environment, you'll be setting the foundation for a lifetime of happiness and health for your child. Enjoy every moment of this incredible adventure.

Sleep and Sleep Training

The journey of parenthood begins with sleepless nights, but with the right approach to sleep and sleep training, fathers can navigate this new chapter successfully. This chapter explores the importance of sleep for both parents and newborns, the challenges faced by first-time dads, and effective strategies for establishing healthy sleep routines for the entire family.

The Importance of Sleep
Sleep is a fundamental human need, and its importance cannot be overstated. Adequate sleep is crucial for physical and mental well-being, as it allows the body to recover, recharge, and consolidate memories. As first-time dads, it's essential to recognize that both parents and newborns require sufficient sleep to thrive.

Challenges Faced by First-Time Dads

First-time dads often encounter unique sleep challenges. The arrival of a newborn disrupts established sleep patterns, leaving fathers feeling sleep-deprived and fatigued. Here are some common challenges faced by new dads:

Irregular Sleep Patterns: Newborns have irregular sleep patterns, waking up frequently during the night for feeding and diaper changes. This disrupts the father's sleep and can lead to exhaustion.

Sleep Deprivation: Consistent sleep deprivation can impact a dad's ability to focus, make decisions, and handle the emotional demands of parenthood.

Adjusting to a New Role: Many first-time dads grapple with the adjustment to their new role as a parent, which can cause anxiety and further disrupt sleep.

Effective Sleep Strategies for First-Time Dads

Teamwork: Parenthood is a shared responsibility. Work as a team with your partner to divide nighttime duties. Taking turns for feedings and diaper changes allows each parent to get some rest.

Create a Sleep-Friendly Environment: Make your baby's sleep environment comfortable and safe. Ensure the room is dimly lit and at a comfortable temperature. White noise machines can help drown out household noises.

Establish a Routine: Babies thrive on routines. Create a bedtime routine that includes activities like bathing, reading, and soothing music. Consistency will signal to your baby that it's time to sleep.

Practise Safe Sleep: Always follow safe sleep guidelines, such as placing your baby on their back to sleep and using a firm mattress in a crib or bassinet.

Take Naps: As a first-time dad, it's crucial to take advantage of opportunities to nap during the day when your baby sleeps. This can help alleviate some of the sleep deprivation.

Seek Support: Don't be afraid to ask for help or advice from experienced parents, friends, or family members. They may have valuable insights on effective sleep training and parenting strategies.

Navigating sleep and sleep training is a significant part of this adventure. Remember that both you and your baby need sufficient sleep for optimal well-being. By working together with your partner and implementing effective sleep strategies, you can create a nurturing environment that promotes healthy sleep patterns for your family. Embrace the joys and challenges of parenthood, knowing that, with time, patience, and love, you will establish a routine that allows everyone to enjoy more peaceful nights.

Feeding and Nutrition

Feeding and nutrition are essential aspects of your child's growth and development, and as a first-time dad, you play a crucial role in their well-being.

One of the first decisions you and your partner will face is whether to breastfeed or use formula. Breast milk is the gold standard for infant nutrition, providing essential nutrients and immune support. However, not all moms can or choose to breastfeed. If breastfeeding isn't an option, modern infant formulas are designed to mimic breast milk's nutritional composition closely.

Understanding your baby's feeding cues is crucial. Babies have tiny stomachs, so they need to eat frequently, typically every 2-3 hours. Watch for signs of hunger like rooting, sucking motions, or increased fussiness. Being attuned to your baby's needs can help you establish a feeding routine.

Around six months, it's time to introduce solid foods. Start with single-ingredient purees like mashed sweet potatoes or peas. As your baby grows, gradually introduce a variety of foods to promote a balanced diet. Keep an eye out for any potential food allergies and consult your paediatrician for guidance.

As your child transitions to solid foods, it's important to provide a balanced diet. Include fruits, vegetables, lean proteins, and whole grains in their meals. Avoid added sugars and excessive salt, and opt for age-appropriate portion sizes. Nutrition sets the foundation for lifelong health.Feeding your child isn't just about nourishment; it's also a bonding experience. Make mealtime enjoyable by sitting face-to-face, making eye contact, and engaging in conversation. This interaction fosters a strong emotional connection with your child.

While it's easy to focus on solid foods, don't forget about hydration. Babies and toddlers need plenty of fluids, primarily breast milk or formula, until they transition to cow's milk at around one year old. Encourage sips of water as your child grows.

Safety is paramount during feeding. Always ensure that food is an appropriate size to prevent choking hazards. Never leave your child unattended while eating, and be cautious with hot foods and liquids.

As a first-time dad, you may have questions or concerns about your child's nutrition. Don't hesitate to consult with healthcare professionals, such as paediatricians or registered dietitians. They can provide personalised guidance based on your child's specific needs.

Parenting is a learning experience, and flexibility is key. Your child's eating habits may change over time. Some days they may be picky eaters, while other days they'll surprise you by trying new foods. Patience and adaptability are your allies.

Lastly, remember that you are your child's role model. Demonstrating healthy eating habits in your own life can influence their choices positively. Share family meals together and make them a cherished part of your daily routine.

Feeding and nutrition are fundamental aspects of parenting for first-time dads. Embrace the journey with enthusiasm and a willingness to learn. Your dedication to providing a nourishing and loving environment will have a lasting impact on your child's health and well-being as they grow.

Health and Safety

The arrival of your newborn is filled with boundless joy and excitement, but it also comes with the profound responsibility of ensuring their health and safety. In this chapter, we will explore essential tips and insights to help you navigate the intricacies of newborn health and safety.

1. Prepare Your Home:
The first step in ensuring your newborn's safety is to create a secure environment at home. Babyproofing your house is paramount. Install safety gates, cover electrical outlets, and secure heavy furniture to prevent accidents. Ensure that smoke detectors and carbon monoxide detectors are functioning correctly. Remove any potential hazards from the baby's reach.

2. Safe Sleep Practices:
Safe sleep is crucial for a newborn's health. The American Academy of Pediatrics recommends that babies sleep on their backs on a firm, flat mattress in a crib or bassinet free of pillows, blankets, or stuffed animals. This reduces the risk of Sudden Infant Death Syndrome (SIDS).

3. Feeding:
Whether you choose to breastfeed or use formula, ensuring your baby is well-fed is essential. Breast milk provides crucial nutrients and boosts the baby's immune system. If you opt for formula, follow the instructions carefully to prepare it safely. Maintain a feeding schedule and monitor your baby's weight gain to ensure they are getting enough nourishment.

4. Hygiene:
Maintaining proper hygiene is paramount for a newborn's health. Wash your hands before handling the baby, and ensure that anyone who touches the baby also follows this practice. Regularly bathe and clean your baby, paying attention to their delicate skin.

5. Immunizations:
Stay up-to-date with your baby's immunization schedule. Vaccines protect your child from potentially life-threatening diseases. Discuss the vaccination schedule

with your paediatrician and address any concerns you may have.

6. Supervision and Interaction:
Newborns require constant supervision. Never leave your baby unattended, especially on elevated surfaces like changing tables. Engage in positive interactions with your baby, including talking, singing, and cuddling. This fosters emotional bonding and stimulates their development.

7. Recognize Signs of Illness:
It's essential to be vigilant and recognize signs of illness in your newborn. Common symptoms include fever, excessive crying, changes in feeding habits, and unusual rashes. Consult your pediatrician if you notice any concerning symptoms.

8. Support for Mom:
Supporting your partner, the baby's mother, is crucial during this time. Encourage her to rest and recover, as her well-being directly

affects the baby's health. Share responsibilities and seek help from family or friends when needed.

9. Educate Yourself:

Continuously educate yourself about newborn care and parenting. Attend parenting classes, read books, and consult reliable sources. Knowledge is a powerful tool in ensuring your baby's health and safety.

10. Trust Your Instincts:

Every baby is unique, and parenting doesn't come with a one-size-fits-all manual. Trust your instincts and the bond you develop with your baby. Be patient, and don't hesitate to seek advice or assistance when uncertain.

By creating a safe environment, practising proper care, and staying informed, you can ensure the health and safety of your precious newborn. Embrace this remarkable chapter of life with love, patience, and unwavering commitment. Your baby is counting on you, and you've got this!

Developmental Milestones

As you hold your precious newborn in your arms, you might find yourself marveling at their tiny fingers and toes, their delicate features, and their seemingly infinite potential. Understanding the developmental milestones of your newborn can help you appreciate the incredible journey of growth and discovery that your little one is embarking upon.

The First Month: A World of Sensory Exploration
In the first few weeks of life, your newborn is primarily focused on adjusting to the world outside the womb. Their senses are in overdrive, and they are learning to adapt to new sensations. During this time, you will notice some significant developmental milestones:

Reflexes: Your baby is born with a set of reflexes that are essential for survival, such as the sucking reflex, which helps them nurse or feed from a bottle.

Eye Contact: While your baby's vision is still blurry, they may begin to make brief eye contact with you, forming the foundation for emotional bonding.

Startle Reflex: Sudden movements or loud noises can trigger the Moro reflex, causing your baby to startle and throw their arms outward.

Social Smiles: Around six weeks, your baby might reward you with their first smile, a heartwarming moment that strengthens the bond between parent and child.

Months 2-3: Growing and Interacting
As your baby enters their second and third months, their development continues at a rapid pace:

Neck Strength: You'll notice improved neck control, allowing your baby to lift their head during tummy time.

Cooing and Gurgling: Your baby will start making delightful cooing sounds, their way of engaging in early communication.

Tracking Objects: Their ability to follow moving objects with their eyes will become more precise.

Grasping: Your baby will begin to explore objects with their hands, albeit with a somewhat clumsy grip.

Months 4-6: Achieving Milestones
Around the 4-6 month mark, your baby will hit some remarkable milestones:

Rolling Over: Many babies begin rolling from tummy to back and vice versa.

Solid Foods: Introducing your baby to solid foods marks a significant step in their development.

Laughter and Babbling: Your baby's laughter and babbling become more frequent and expressive.

Sitting Up: With improved muscle strength, your baby may start sitting with support.

Months 7-12: Active Explorers
During this period, your baby transforms into an active explorer:

Crawling: Some babies begin crawling, while others opt for scooting or bottom shuffling.

First Words: Expect to hear their first words, usually simple sounds like "mama" and "dada."

Standing with Support: Your baby may pull themselves up to a standing position with the help of furniture.

Pincer Grasp: Fine motor skills progress, allowing them to pick up small objects with their thumb and forefinger.

Social Awareness: Your baby will show a growing interest in other people, making connections with family members and caregivers.

Celebrating Every Step
As a first-time dad, it's essential to remember that every child develops at their own pace. While these milestones provide a general guideline, some babies may reach them earlier or later. What's most important is to cherish each moment of your baby's journey and offer them love, care, and support as they grow and explore the world around them. Parenthood is an incredible adventure, and watching your child reach

these developmental milestones is a rewarding part of that journey. Enjoy every step of it!

Parenting Roles and Relationships

One of the most crucial aspects of this journey is understanding and establishing parenting roles and relationships, especially with a newborn. In this chapter, we'll explore the multifaceted world of first-time fatherhood and offer valuable insights into nurturing your relationship with your newborn.

The Role of a First-Time Dad
As a first-time dad, your role in your newborn's life is irreplaceable. While traditionally, parenting roles might have been more rigid, today's fathers are encouraged to be actively involved from the very beginning. Here are some key aspects of your role:

a. Providing Emotional Support: Your newborn may not understand words, but they can feel your love and presence. Comforting, cuddling, and being emotionally available are vital in building a strong bond.

b. Sharing Responsibilities: Changing diapers, helping with feedings, and participating in daily routines can deepen your connection with your baby and relieve some of the burdens on your partner.

c. Being Patient and Flexible: Newborns have unpredictable schedules, and patience is key. Be adaptable, as your baby's needs and routines can change frequently.

Building a Strong Relationship with Your Newborn.
The early days with a newborn can be both rewarding and challenging. Here's how you can build a strong relationship with your baby:

a. Skin-to-Skin Contact: Holding your baby skin-to-skin promotes bonding, regulates their temperature, and provides a sense of security.

b. Talk and Sing: Babies love hearing their parents' voices. Engage in baby talk, sing lullabies, or simply narrate what you're doing. This helps develop their language skills and creates a sense of familiarity.

c. Eye Contact: Locking eyes with your newborn during feedings and cuddles can be profoundly meaningful. It's a way to communicate love and trust without words.
d. Read to Your Baby: Even though they can't understand the story, reading aloud introduces your child to the rhythm of language and sets the stage for future literacy.

Nurturing Your Relationship with Your Partner,Maintaining a strong relationship with your partner is equally important during this period.

a. Communicate Openly: Parenthood can be challenging, and you'll both experience moments of stress. Open and honest communication is essential for understanding each other's needs and feelings.

b. Share Responsibilities: Divide household and baby care tasks to ensure that both partners have time for self-care and couple time.
c. Support Each Other: Acknowledge the unique challenges and joys each of you experiences as new parents. Support each other emotionally and physically.

By actively participating in parenting roles, nurturing your baby's development, and maintaining a strong partnership with your spouse, you can embark on this journey with confidence and love. Remember, your presence and dedication are invaluable in shaping your child's future and fostering a loving family environment.

Financial Planning

Another aspect that can contribute significantly to your peace of mind during this transformative journey is financial planning. Welcoming a new member into your family means more than just changing diapers and late-night feedings; it means taking proactive steps to secure your child's future while managing the present. In this chapter, we'll explore the essential elements of financial planning for first-time dads.

*Set Clear Financial Goals:*The foundation of any effective financial plan is setting clear, achievable goals. As a new dad, your goals may include saving for your child's education, creating an emergency fund, buying a larger home, or simply ensuring your family's financial security. Write down your goals and prioritize them to create a roadmap for your financial journey.

*Create a Budget:*Budgeting is the cornerstone of sound financial planning. Track your income and expenses to understand where your money goes. Make adjustments to cut unnecessary spending and allocate more towards your financial goals. Remember that every dollar saved today can have a substantial impact on your child's future.

*Build an Emergency Fund:*Unexpected expenses can arise at any time. Building an emergency fund equivalent to three to six months' worth of living expenses can provide a safety net during challenging times, such as medical emergencies or job loss.

*Life Insurance:*Protect your family's financial future by investing in life insurance. Ensure that your coverage is sufficient to cover your outstanding debts, mortgage, and provide financial stability to your family in your absence.

*Start Saving for Education:*College tuition costs continue to rise. Consider opening a 529 savings plan or a similar education savings account to prepare for your child's future educational expenses. The earlier you start, the more time your money has to grow.

*Invest Wisely:*Investing is a powerful tool for growing your wealth over the long term. Diversify your investments to spread risk, and consider consulting a financial advisor to create an investment strategy tailored to your family's goals.

*Plan for Retirement:*While it may seem distant, planning for retirement is crucial. A well-funded retirement account will ensure you're not a financial burden on your children when you're older. Maximize contributions to employer-sponsored retirement plans and explore other retirement investment options.

*Estate Planning:*Draft a will to ensure your assets are distributed according to your wishes in case of unforeseen events. Designate a guardian for your child, and consider creating a trust to manage and protect assets for their future.

Review and Adjust:Life circumstances change, and so should your financial plan. Periodically review and adjust your goals, budget, and investment strategy to align with your family's evolving needs.

*Seek Professional Advice:*Financial planning can be complex, and it's okay to seek help. A financial advisor can provide valuable insights, help you make informed decisions, and guide you toward your goals.

As a first-time dad, your responsibility extends beyond providing love and care for your child. It encompasses ensuring their financial well-being and security. By following these steps and committing to a comprehensive financial plan, you'll not only navigate parenthood with confidence but also lay the groundwork for a prosperous future for your family. Remember, the most precious gift you can give your child is a stable and secure financial foundation.

Emotional Support

While much attention is rightly given to the physical aspects of pregnancy and childbirth, the emotional support provided by fathers during this transformative period is equally crucial. In this chapter, we'll explore the role of emotional support for first-time dads, the impact it has on their partners, and the benefits it brings to the entire family.

As a first-time dad, you embark on a rollercoaster of emotions. Excitement, anticipation, and even anxiety are all part of the package. Witnessing the physical and emotional changes in your partner can be both thrilling and daunting. It's essential to recognize that your emotional well-being matters just as much as your partner's during this time.

Empathy is the cornerstone of emotional support. Taking the time to understand your partner's experiences, concerns, and fears can create a stronger emotional bond. Attend prenatal classes together, read books on pregnancy, and engage in open conversations about your expectations as parents. This will not only strengthen your relationship but also help you better prepare for parenthood.One of the most powerful forms of emotional support is simply being present. Attend doctor's appointments and ultrasounds, hold her hand during labor, and be the shoulder she can lean on when things get tough. Your physical presence can provide immense comfort and reassurance.

Effective communication is a vital tool for emotional support. Create a safe space where your partner feels comfortable expressing her thoughts and feelings. Sometimes, all she needs is someone to listen without judgment. Encourage open dialogue, share your own thoughts and concerns, and work together to find solutions to any challenges that arise.

As a first-time dad, actively participating in household and baby-related tasks demonstrates your commitment to shared responsibility. This not only eases the burden on your partner but also fosters a sense of teamwork and togetherness. Changing diapers, preparing meals, and taking turns with nighttime feedings are all opportunities to bond with your child and support your partner.

Remember that taking care of your own emotional well-being is essential for providing effective support. It's okay to feel overwhelmed at times. Seek support from friends, family, or even professional counseling if needed. Maintaining a healthy work-life balance and finding moments to relax and recharge will enable you to be the best partner and father you can be.

Emotional support for first-time dads doesn't only benefit you and your partner; it has a profound ripple effect on your child and the entire family. Children thrive in environments where their parents are emotionally connected and supportive. By nurturing a strong emotional foundation, you contribute to your child's sense of security and well-being.

Emotional support is a cornerstone of successful fatherhood for first-time dads. By actively engaging in your partner's pregnancy journey, practising empathy and open communication, and sharing responsibilities, you not only strengthen your relationship but also create a nurturing environment for your child to grow. The journey into fatherhood is a shared adventure, and the power of emotional support will guide you through its beautiful ups and downs.

Father-Child Bonding

Among the countless changes that parenthood brings, the father-child bond is one of the most precious and rewarding aspects of this journey. In this chapter, we will explore the enchanting and heartwarming process of bonding between a first-time dad and his child.

For a first-time dad, the first encounter with their newborn child is nothing short of magical. Holding that tiny bundle of joy in their arms for the first time, feeling the warmth of their child's skin, and gazing into their innocent eyes are moments that etch themselves into a father's heart forever. It's a surreal experience that leaves dads in awe of the miracle of life and ignites an unbreakable connection.

As a first-time dad, the power of touch becomes your most potent tool for bonding. Skin-to-skin contact, in particular, is a beautiful and intimate way to connect with your baby. It's not just about providing warmth; it's about establishing trust and security. Babies feel their father's heartbeat, and this rhythm can be incredibly soothing, reminding the child of the safety and comfort that only a father's embrace can provide.

In the early months, your child may not yet speak words, but the two of you will begin communicating in your own unique language. The coos, giggles, and gurgles of your baby will be music to your ears. Responding to these sounds with your own laughter and soothing words will create a special bond built on trust and understanding. Over time, you will learn to interpret your child's cues, understanding their needs even before they can express them.As a first-time dad, your child will relish the time you spend together. Whether it's reading a bedtime story, playing peek-a-boo, or simply cuddling on the couch, these moments are where the magic happens. Your child will look up to you as their hero, and every shared experience becomes a building block in your evolving relationship.

One of the most important roles a first-time dad plays is that of a mentor and guide. As your child grows, you will be there to support them through their first steps, their first words, and all the firsts that life has to offer. Your unwavering presence and encouragement will help shape your child's self-esteem and confidence.Every interaction, every shared smile, and every comforting hug adds to the tapestry of memories that you and your child will weave together. These memories will form the foundation of your relationship and serve as a source of strength and comfort in the years to come.

A Bond That Grows Stronger with Time
The bond between a father and child is a treasure that deepens with each passing day, creating a lifelong connection that is as enduring as it is beautiful. As a first-time dad, you have the privilege of witnessing your child's growth and being a source of

love and support throughout their life. Cherish these moments, for they are the building blocks of a bond that will stand the test of time.

Discipline and Boundaries

As you embark on this incredible journey, it's essential to recognize the pivotal role that discipline and boundaries play in your child's upbringing. These fundamental aspects of parenting are the compass guiding you through the challenges and triumphs of fatherhood.

Before diving into the practicalities, let's define these terms.

Discipline refers to the process of teaching your child appropriate behaviors, values, and self-control. It's not about punishment but rather nurturing positive character traits. Boundaries, on the other hand, are the limits you set for your child, helping them understand what's acceptable and safe. Together, discipline and boundaries create a secure and structured environment for your child to grow.

One of the first things you'll learn as a new dad is that consistency is crucial. Children thrive in predictable environments where they know what to expect. Set consistent rules and consequences, and stick to them. Whether it's bedtime routines, mealtime behavior, or playtime limits, be unwavering in your approach.

Children are like sponges, absorbing everything around them, especially from their parents. As a first-time dad, you are your child's first role model. Show them the values and behaviors you want them to emulate. If you want your child to be polite, respectful, and kind, demonstrate these qualities in your interactions with them and others.

Communication is the cornerstone of discipline and setting boundaries. Explain to your child why certain rules exist and the consequences of breaking them. Use age-appropriate language, so they can understand. Encourage questions and open dialogues. This not only helps them comprehend the importance of boundaries but also strengthens the parent-child bond.

While consistency is essential, it's also vital to be flexible within the established boundaries. As your child grows, their needs and abilities change. Be prepared to adapt your approach accordingly. What worked when they were toddlers may not be suitable for preschoolers or teenagers. Flexibility allows you to nurture their independence while maintaining a safe environment.
Remember to celebrate your child's successes and positive behaviors. Praise and rewards can be powerful motivators. When they adhere to the boundaries and demonstrate good behavior, acknowledge it. This positive reinforcement encourages them to continue making wise choices.Parenthood is a learning journey for both you and your child. Don't be too hard on yourself when you make mistakes. Instead, view them as opportunities to grow and adapt your parenting style. Seek advice

from experienced parents, read parenting books, or attend parenting classes. The willingness to learn and evolve is a testament to your dedication as a dad.

As a first-time dad, embracing discipline and boundaries is a cornerstone of your child's upbringing. It provides the structure and guidance they need to develop into responsible, well-adjusted individuals. Remember, parenting is a marathon, not a sprint. Your unwavering love, consistent discipline, and healthy boundaries will be the compass guiding your child through life's ups and downs, helping them become the best version of themselves.

Parenting Styles

As you embark on this adventure, one of the most crucial aspects to consider is your parenting style. Your approach to parenting will shape your child's development, so it's essential to explore the various styles and find what works best for you and your family.

Authoritarian Parenting:
This parenting style is characterized by strict rules and high expectations. Authoritarian parents prioritize discipline and obedience, often using punishments for rule violations. While structure and boundaries are crucial, it's essential to balance them with warmth and understanding. As a first-time dad, you may find yourself leaning toward this style initially, especially if you want to maintain order in your home. However, remember that fostering open communication and empathy is equally important.

Permissive Parenting:
Permissive parents tend to be lenient and indulgent, allowing their children significant freedom without many rules or consequences. While it's vital to be flexible and give your child room to explore,

excessive permissiveness can lead to a lack of boundaries. As a first-time dad, finding a balance between granting freedom and setting appropriate limits is key. It's essential to provide guidance while respecting your child's individuality.

Authoritative Parenting:
Authoritative parenting strikes a balance between discipline and warmth. Parents in this category set clear expectations and boundaries but also encourage independence and open communication. As a first-time dad, aiming for an authoritative approach can be beneficial. It fosters a healthy parent-child relationship built on mutual respect and trust, setting a positive foundation for your child's development.

Uninvolved Parenting:
Uninvolved parenting, as the name suggests, involves minimal emotional involvement and supervision. Parents who follow this style may provide basic necessities but often

neglect their child's emotional needs. As a first-time dad, it's essential to be engaged and present in your child's life. Emotional support and active participation are crucial for their overall well-being.

Helicopter Parenting:
Helicopter parents tend to be overly involved and excessively protective. They hover over their children, making decisions and solving problems for them. While it's natural to want to protect your child, it's essential to allow them to learn from their experiences and mistakes. As a first-time dad, resist the urge to hover too closely. Encourage independence and problem-solving skills, which are vital for their development.

Free-Range Parenting:
Free-range parenting encourages independence and self-sufficiency in children. Parents who follow this style allow their kids to explore the world with minimal

intervention. While independence is valuable, it's crucial to strike a balance between giving your child freedom and ensuring their safety. As a first-time dad, it's your responsibility to provide guidance and monitor your child's activities, all while fostering their independence.

As you explore these different parenting styles, remember that there is no one-size-fits-all approach. Every child is unique, and your parenting style may evolve as you get to know your child better. The key is to adapt and find a balance that supports your child's development while maintaining a loving and nurturing environment. Parenthood is an ongoing journey of discovery, and being open to change and growth is the most important style of all.

Preparing for Future Stages

As you prepare to welcome your new addition to the family, it's essential to not only focus on the present but also look ahead to future stages of your child's development. Here's a comprehensive guide on how to prepare for the future stages as a first-time dad.

Knowledge is your best ally in fatherhood. Begin by reading books, attending parenting classes, or seeking advice from experienced fathers. Understanding child development, from infancy to adolescence, will help you anticipate your child's needs and challenges.Parenthood comes with financial responsibilities. Start budgeting and saving for your child's future education and other expenses. Consider setting up a college fund or investment account to secure their future.

Don't hesitate to lean on friends, family, and fellow dads for support and advice. Connect with other first-time fathers through parenting groups or online forums. Sharing experiences and seeking guidance from those who've been through it can be invaluable.

As your child grows, so does their curiosity. Baby-proofing your home is an ongoing process. Begin with the basics, like covering electrical outlets and securing cabinets, and adapt as your child starts crawling and walking.
Your child's future depends on your well-being. Maintain a healthy lifestyle, including a balanced diet and regular exercise. Prioritize your mental health too; being emotionally available for your child is essential.

Parenthood can put strain on relationships. Communicate openly with your partner about your expectations and fears. Make time for each other and keep the romance alive to strengthen your bond as parents.

It's never too early to think about your child's education. Research educational options in your area and start saving for their schooling. Stay involved in their learning journey as they grow.
Beyond academics, teach your child important life skills such as problem-solving, empathy, and communication. These skills will serve them well in their future stages of development.

As your child grows, encourage their independence. Let them make age-appropriate decisions and learn from their experiences. This will help them become self-reliant individuals.

Be prepared for the constant changes that come with parenting. Children grow, develop, and evolve, and your role as a dad will adapt accordingly. Stay flexible and open to new challenges.
Make a conscious effort to spend quality time with your child. Create lasting

memories through family outings, activities, and traditions that will shape their future and strengthen your bond.As your child discovers their interests and talents, support and encourage their passions. Whether it's sports, music, art, or academics, nurturing their talents can pave the way for future success.

Be the role model your child needs. Demonstrate kindness, respect, and responsibility in your actions, as your child will emulate your behavior in their future interactions.

Keep yourself informed about the latest parenting trends, technologies, and resources. The world is evolving, and staying updated will help you adapt to the changing needs of your child.Most importantly, savor every moment of fatherhood. Children grow up faster than you think, so relish the joy and wonder they bring to your life at every stage.

By preparing for the future stages, you can ensure that you're ready to support your child in their development and create a bright and promising future for them. Embrace this role with enthusiasm and cherish the precious moments with your little one along the way.

Self-Care

One often overlooked but essential aspect is self-care. In the whirlwind of diaper changes, sleepless nights, and soothing lullabies, taking care of yourself is paramount for both you and your growing family.

The Importance of Self-Care
Self-care isn't selfish; it's self-preservation. Think of it as the oxygen mask on an airplane - before you can assist others, you must secure your mask first. As a new dad, you'll be taking on a multitude of responsibilities, and being at your best physically and mentally is crucial.

Sleep Matters
In those initial months, sleep may seem like a luxury. However, prioritizing rest is essential. When the baby sleeps, consider taking a nap. Share nighttime duties with your partner to ensure you both get enough

sleep. Chronic sleep deprivation can impact your mood, cognitive function, and overall well-being.

Balanced Diet

Maintaining a balanced diet is not only for the baby but for you too. Eating nutritious meals provides you with the energy needed to tackle the demands of parenthood. Try to have quick, healthy snacks on hand to keep your energy levels stable during those hectic days.

Exercise

Exercise isn't just for sculpting your beach body; it's also a fantastic stress-reliever. Even a short daily walk or some light stretches can do wonders for your mental and physical health. Plus, it gives you a break from the baby duties and some time to clear your mind.

Connect with Others

Being a dad can sometimes feel isolating, especially if you're the only one in your social circle with a newborn. Reach out to fellow dads, join parenting groups, or simply have a chat with a friend. Sharing experiences and concerns can provide much-needed emotional support.

Carve Out "Me" Time

Don't forget to set aside time for yourself. Whether it's reading a book, watching your favorite show, or pursuing a hobby, having moments to recharge is crucial. This can also strengthen your relationship with your partner, as you both get a chance to miss each other and cherish your time together.

Communicate with Your Partner

Open and honest communication with your partner is key. Share your feelings, concerns, and aspirations. Support each other in your self-care routines, and work as a team to navigate the challenges of parenthood.

Seek Professional Help if Needed
If you find yourself overwhelmed, anxious, or struggling with your mental health, don't hesitate to seek professional help. A therapist or counselor can provide guidance and support during this transformative time.

By taking care of yourself physically and mentally, you're not only ensuring your well-being but also setting a positive example for your child. Remember, self-care isn't a luxury; it's a necessity. So, embrace it, and savor every moment of this incredible adventure called fatherhood.

Community and Resources

As you step into this new role, you'll quickly realize that you're not alone. There's a vast and supportive community of fellow first-time dads and an abundance of resources to help you navigate this incredible adventure.

One of the most reassuring aspects of becoming a first-time dad is that you're not the only one going through it. Joining a dad-to-dad community can be incredibly beneficial for emotional support and sharing experiences. These communities often exist both online and in person, offering a safe space to discuss your concerns, fears, and joys. Online forums, social media groups, and local dad clubs are excellent places to start building your network.

Diving into the world of parenthood literature can be enlightening. There are countless blogs and books written by experienced fathers who share their wisdom, anecdotes, and advice. From humorous takes on diaper-changing mishaps to heartfelt stories of bonding with your child, these resources can provide valuable insights and a sense of camaraderie.

Attending parenting classes can equip you with practical knowledge on subjects like baby care, childbirth, and infant CPR. These classes often include group discussions, which can lead to lasting friendships with other first-time dads who are eager to learn just like you.
In the digital age, there's an app for everything, including parenting. Many apps are designed specifically for new fathers, offering advice, tracking tools, and even forums to connect with other dads. These apps can be a convenient resource for on-the-go dads who want to stay engaged and informed.

Your loved ones are often eager to provide guidance and support during this transformative time. Don't hesitate to reach out to experienced friends, family members, or coworkers who have been through parenthood. Their personal experiences and advice can be invaluable.

If you're feeling overwhelmed or struggling with the demands of fatherhood, seeking professional help is a courageous step. Therapists, counselors, and support groups are available to address any emotional challenges you may encounter.

In addition to local dad groups, numerous online communities offer a platform for fathers to connect. Websites, social media, and forums provide a space for discussing everything from sleepless nights to baby gear recommendations. Engaging with these online communities can provide a sense of belonging and a wealth of knowledge.

A thriving community of fellow fathers, coupled with a wide range of resources, ensures that you have the support and knowledge you need to embrace fatherhood with confidence. Whether you connect with other dads at local meetups or seek advice from parenting blogs, remember that you're part of a community that celebrates the incredible journey of parenthood. Embrace it, learn from it, and cherish every moment as a first-time dad.

Balancing Work and Parenting

One of the most significant challenges new fathers face is finding the delicate equilibrium between their professional responsibilities and the demands of parenting. In this chapter, we'll delve into the art of balancing work and parenting, offering valuable insights and practical tips for first-time dads embarking on this transformative journey.

As a first-time dad, it's crucial to accept that your life is about to become more dynamic than ever before. Flexibility will be your greatest ally. Understand that your daily routine may undergo unpredictable changes, especially during the initial months when your baby's sleep patterns are erratic. Embracing this flexibility will help you navigate the challenges that lie ahead.

Open and honest communication with your employer is vital when balancing work and parenting. Inform them of your new responsibilities and any potential schedule adjustments you may need. Many companies are accommodating and willing to work with new parents to find a suitable balance. Establishing clear expectations can reduce stress and ensure a smoother transition.

Remember that parenting is a shared responsibility. Support and communication with your partner are key to maintaining a harmonious household. Discuss and delegate tasks, share the baby-related duties, and ensure you're both on the same page regarding your parenting goals and values. A united front makes parenting more manageable.

Efficient time management becomes your lifeline when balancing work and parenting. Prioritize tasks and create a schedule that accommodates both work and family time. Utilize tools like calendars and to-do lists to stay organized. Be prepared to adapt your schedule as your baby's needs evolve.

You don't have to do it all alone. Don't hesitate to seek help from family, friends, or professional services when necessary. A supportive network can provide much-needed relief and guidance, allowing you to recharge and maintain your well-being.

When spending time with your child, focus on quality over quantity. Engage in meaningful interactions that foster bonding and development. Put away distractions like smartphones and fully immerse yourself in those precious moments with your little one. Remember that taking care of yourself is essential for being a great parent. Prioritize self-care, including proper sleep, nutrition, and exercise. Finding moments for relaxation and personal hobbies can help you recharge, ensuring you're in the best shape to care for your family.

It's crucial to set realistic expectations for both your work and parenting roles. Understand that perfection is unattainable, and there will be challenging days. Be kind to yourself and celebrate small victories along the way.

Balancing work and parenting as a first-time dad is an ongoing journey filled with learning experiences. By embracing flexibility, effective communication, time management, and self-care, you can navigate this new chapter in your life successfully. Remember that every moment you spend with your child is precious, and your efforts to balance these roles will contribute to a loving and fulfilling family life.

Travelling with a Baby

The journey into fatherhood is an incredible adventure filled with countless firsts, and one of the most exciting and nerve-wracking experiences for a first-time dad is travelling with a baby. Whether it's a weekend getaway or a cross-country road trip, embarking on these adventures with your little one can be both rewarding and challenging. In this article, we'll explore the world of travelling with a baby from a first-time dad's perspective, offering insights, tips, and heartwarming anecdotes that capture the essence of this unique journey.

Preparing for the Journey
The key to a successful trip with a baby starts with meticulous planning. As a first-time dad, it's essential to create a detailed itinerary, packing list, and contingency plan for unexpected situations. This preparation will give you confidence as you embark on your adventure.

Babies come with a long list of essentials, from diapers and wipes to baby food and toys. Make sure to pack these necessities and always have a few extras on hand. Don't forget a well-stocked diaper bag for on-the-go changes.

Selecting the right mode of transportation is crucial. For long trips, consider whether a road trip, train journey, or a flight is the most convenient option for your family. Each has its own set of challenges and advantages.

Babies thrive on routine and comfort. Bring along their favorite blanket or stuffed animal to provide a sense of security, especially during travel. Ensure the car seat or stroller is comfortable and correctly installed.

Babies require frequent breaks for feeding, changing, and playtime. Factor in extra time for these stops during your journey. It's a chance to bond with your baby and relieve some of their restlessness.

A variety of baby-friendly entertainment is essential to keep your little one occupied. Consider soft books, toys that make soothing sounds, or even a tablet with age-appropriate content.

Babies need their sleep, and travel can disrupt their usual routine. Be prepared to adapt and find creative solutions to help your baby nap or sleep peacefully on the go. A portable crib or a comfortable baby carrier can be a lifesaver.

If your baby is breastfed, consider nursing during breaks. For formula-fed babies, bring pre-measured formula and a bottle warmer. Solid foods can be trickier, so opt for easy-to-prepare and mess-free options.

Travelling with your baby as a first-time dad creates countless precious moments. Don't forget to capture these memories through photos and videos. They will be cherished reminders of this unique experience.

Travelling with your baby fosters a strong bond and allows you to witness their growth firsthand. Each new experience, from their first taste of beach sand to their awe at seeing new landscapes, is a testament to the joy of parenthood.

Travelling with a baby as a first-time dad is an adventure filled with challenges and rewards. It's an opportunity to create lasting memories, strengthen your bond with your child, and gain confidence as a parent. With careful planning, adaptability, and a sense of adventure, you'll discover that the world is full of wonders waiting to be explored together, one journey at a time.

Creating Memories

Becoming a father for the first time is a profound and life-altering experience. It's a journey filled with a rollercoaster of emotions, sleepless nights, and the overwhelming feeling of responsibility. However, amid the chaos and diapers, there are those magical moments that define fatherhood and create lasting memories.

The First Glimpse: The moment your child is born is an indescribable mix of awe, joy, and nervousness. As a first-time dad, seeing your newborn for the first time is an overwhelming experience. The tiny, fragile life you've helped bring into the world becomes an instant source of inspiration and love.

The Midnight Lullabies: Those late-night feedings and diaper changes can be exhausting, but they also offer a unique bonding opportunity. As you hold your baby in the dimly lit room, singing soft lullabies or gently rocking them to sleep, you create a connection that goes beyond words. It's in these quiet moments that you become a source of comfort and security.

The First Smile: One of the most heartwarming moments as a new dad is witnessing your baby's first smile. That radiant, toothless grin that lights up their face is an affirmation of your role as a parent. It's a sign that your baby recognizes you and feels happiness in your presence.

Exploring the World Together: As your child grows, you'll have countless opportunities to explore the world together. Whether it's taking your baby for their first walk in the park, visiting the zoo, or simply introducing them to the wonders of nature in your backyard, these adventures become cherished memories.

Teaching Moments: From teaching your child to tie their shoes to helping them with their homework, every moment spent imparting knowledge is a gift. As a first-time dad, you're not just a caretaker but also a guide, imparting valuable life lessons and watching your child grow and learn.

The Unpredictable Laughter: Babies have an uncanny ability to find humor in the simplest things. Whether it's a peek-a-boo game, a funny face you make, or a silly noise, the sound of your baby's infectious laughter will bring immeasurable joy to your heart.

Bedtime Stories: Reading bedtime stories to your child is a tradition cherished by many fathers. The excitement in your child's eyes as they listen to your voice weaving tales of adventure and imagination is a memory that both of you will treasure.

First Steps and Milestones: Watching your baby take their first steps is a monumental moment. Those tentative wobbles and giggles of accomplishment are a testament to your support and encouragement. Celebrating milestones like the first word, the first tooth, and the first day of school are all part of the incredible journey of fatherhood.

Daddy-Daughter or Daddy-Son Days: Special days spent with your child one-on-one create enduring bonds. Whether it's a father-daughter dance, a father-son fishing trip, or a day at the amusement park, these moments are etched in your child's memory as they grow older.

The Hugs and "I Love Yous": Never underestimate the power of a hug or an "I love you" shared with your child. These small gestures carry immense weight and reassure your child of your love and support.

As a first-time dad, you embark on a journey filled with wonder and love. While there will be challenges along the way, the moments of joy, connection, and love will far outweigh them. These precious moments will shape not only your child's life but also your own, making you a better, stronger, and more loving father with each passing day. So savor every second, for time flies, and these moments are the building blocks of a beautiful father-child relationship.

Conclusion

Becoming a first-time dad is a remarkable journey filled with a multitude of emotions, challenges, and heartwarming moments. It's a transition that reshapes one's life in ways previously unimaginable. As we reach the conclusion of this exploration into the world of first-time fatherhood, it's essential to reflect on the profound transformation that occurs in a man's life when he embraces this role.

First and foremost, the journey into fatherhood is a deeply personal one. From the moment you hold your newborn in your arms, you're forever changed. The sleepless nights, diaper changes, and endless feedings become a labor of love, and you quickly realize that your capacity for patience, empathy, and selflessness grows exponentially.

One of the most significant takeaways from the experience of being a first-time dad is the newfound appreciation for the fragility and resilience of life. Witnessing a tiny, vulnerable human being develop and thrive under your care is both awe-inspiring and humbling. It teaches you to cherish every moment and find joy in the simple things, like your baby's first smile or their small victories along the way.

Furthermore, becoming a father introduces you to a unique brand of love—a love that is boundless, unconditional, and selfless. It's a love that transcends words and can only be truly understood when experienced. This love forms an unbreakable bond between you and your child, forging a connection that will shape their development and your own for years to come.

On the flip side, fatherhood comes with its fair share of challenges. Balancing work, personal life, and the responsibilities of being a parent can be daunting. The sleep deprivation and occasional feelings of inadequacy are real, but they are outweighed by the joy and fulfillment that parenthood brings.

Ultimately, being a first-time dad is a transformative journey that teaches you about love, resilience, and the incredible capacity of the human heart. It's about guiding, nurturing, and supporting a new life while discovering new dimensions of yourself in the process. The path is far from linear, but the rewards are immeasurable.

In conclusion, the adventure of becoming a first-time dad is a rollercoaster of emotions, challenges, and growth. It's about embracing the messy, beautiful chaos of parenthood and finding profound meaning in the everyday moments. It's a journey that reshapes your identity, redefines your priorities, and fills your heart with a love like no other. So, to all the first-time dads embarking on this incredible voyage, cherish every step, for it's a journey that will shape your life in ways you never thought possible.